Keto Chaffle

Recipes

Cookbook

The Ultimate Cookbook For Weight Loss And Boost Metabolism

Diana Humble

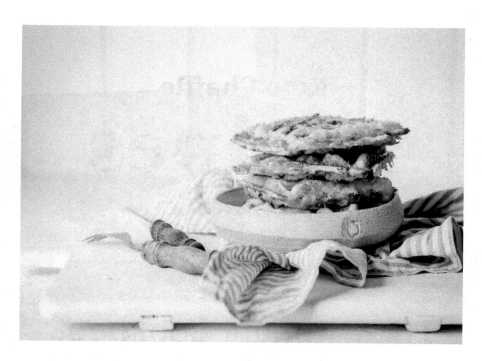

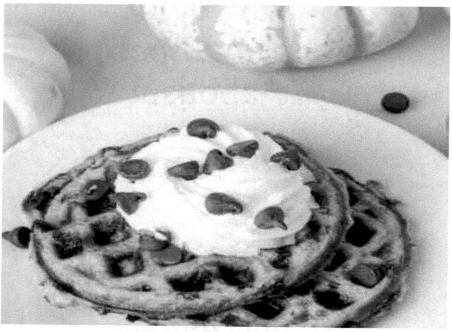

TABLE OF CONTENTS

allowed with the express written consent from the Publisher. All additional right reserved.

The information in the following pages is broadly considered a truthful and accurate account of facts and as such, any inattention, use, or misuse of the information in question by the reader will render any resulting actions solely under their purview. There are no scenarios in which the publisher or the original author of this work can be in any fashion deemed liable for any hardship or damages that may befall them after undertaking information described herein.

Additionally, the information in the following pages is intended only for informational purposes and should thus be thought of as universal. As befitting its nature, it is presented without assurance regarding its prolonged validity or interim quality. Trademarks that are mentioned are done without written consent and can in no way be considered an endorsement from the trademark holder.

INTRODUCTION

Keto Diet is a high-fat, low-carb diet that is an increasingly popular way to lose weight. Keto is short for "ketosis", which occurs when the body has depleted its sugar stores, so it burns stored fat instead of glucose in order to produce energy.

Losing weight on a keto diet sounds pretty easy; just eat a few bacon sandwiches and you'll be slimmer in no time. However, there are drawbacks to this diet, including very low levels of vegetables and fruit (so important for fiber and other nutrients) as well as constipation from lack of dietary fiber. Here are some tips:

- It's important to drink plenty of water, not only because you may be eating more sodium than you need, but because staying hydrated will help your body process proteins and fats more efficiently.

- For best results, stay away from most fruits and vegetables. Some berries are allowed; others aren't. Vegetables that are considered "low in carbs" or "leafy greens" are fine—but there is a difference between low-carb and high-fiber. As a rule of thumb, if it looks like it has the texture of tree bark or is covered with seeds or bulbs (e.g., artichokes), it probably has a lot of carbs and should be avoided.

- Be careful with spices, which tend to have a lot of sugar; salt is OK. It can be easy to go overboard on spices.

- Eat plenty of salmon, tuna and egg whites. Meat—including beef, chicken, pork and lamb—should comprise 20 to 25 percent of your total diet. (Be aware that "lean" meat is often not very lean. Be prepared to trim off most of that fat before cooking.) A little bacon or sausage is fine, too.

- Avoid condiments and sauces, including barbecue sauce and ketchup. These are full of sugar and other unhealthy ingredients.

- Drink mostly water (or unsweetened drinks such as tea or coffee). Try to avoid drinks with a lot of added sugar, like fruit juice or alcohol. If you choose to drink wine, go for the dry stuff—red wine is best.

Now, for Chaffles.

What is Chaffle?

Keto chaffle recipe is a versatile and easy-to-make low carb pancake that only requires 2 ingredients. It's a way to satisfy your sweet cravings while staying keto!

Chaffle is made from cheese and eggs. You will need grated cheddar cheese (use any kind of cheese you have on hand) and eggs, beaten together, then fried in a pan with butter or coconut oil.

Chaffles are perfect for a low carb breakfast, lunch or dinner and can be a treat right out of the pan, with butter!

Why Keto and Chaffle is a perfect combination?

Keto Chaffle is a great way to satisfy your sweet cravings while staying 100% in ketosis. It helps you feel fuller for longer but at the same time it's not a high carb treat.

Chaffle gives you a lot of energy and it's an easy way to prepare breakfast if you want it to be ready quickly when you get up or even if you're in a hurry so it can be prepared on the go without any issues.

Keto Chaffle tastes amazing plain, with butter or with any toppings you like and it can also be used as sandwich bread substitute.

KETOGENIC DIET AND ITS BENEFITS

What is Ketogenic Diet?

The ketogenic diet is a low-carb, high-fat diet. This means that the macronutrient ratio of your diet should consist mainly of fat and protein with only a small percentage of carbohydrates.

The idea behind the ketogenic diet is to force your body to use fat rather than glucose as its primary fuel source. When we are in ketosis, we can function on almost any fuel source.

Benefits of the Ketogenic Diet

The benefits of the ketogenic diet are as follows:

1. No need to count calories.

On this diet, you can eat as much as you want. Since there are no grains, the carbohydrates in the diet are very low, and so you will not take in many calories.

2. There is no need to spend a lot of money on expensive foods.

Since this diet is high in fat, one of the cheapest sources of fat is chicken thighs and legs and other skinless poultry parts or meats from around the animal, such as organ meats (heart, liver, etc.).

3. Low levels of Beta-hydroxybutyrate (ketone body) is suitable for brain health

The ketogenic diet can increase the level of ketone bodies by 10 times than normal dietary levels through fat metabolism.

4. Decreased risk of heart disease

Many people can lower their LDL (bad) cholesterol by 75-90% and triglyceride levels by 60%.

5. Less inflammation

Because there are no carbohydrates in the ketogenic diet, your body becomes very efficient at burning ketones as fuel. This is excellent news if you have an autoimmune disorder like rheumatoid arthritis or Crohn's disease because inflammation is often linked to autoimmune problems.

6. Fast weight loss

People usually start losing weight within two weeks of starting the diet.

7. Increased energy levels

The ketogenic diet can increase your energy levels because you will be consuming a high-fat diet with very few carbohydrates.

8. No constant hunger

When people are on a ketogenic diet, they are in "ketosis." This means that their bodies are using fat as an almost complete fuel source. This is the opposite of how most people function in a non-ketogenic state, which usually involves using carbohydrates (sugars) as a practically whole fuel source. Because the ketogenic diet is so different, the body is forced to use fat as its primary fuel source to function. This means you won't be hungry all the time once you get the hang of it.

9. No need for cheat meals

Since carbohydrates are reduced in this diet, cheating on the ketogenic diet will not help you lose weight because your body does not have carbohydrates stored to keep your metabolism running, being that fat is used instead of sugar/carbs.

10. No need to buy expensive supplements

Since the diet is not very restrictive, you won't need to buy many supplements besides vitamin D3 if you are deficient.

11. You can gain muscle and lose fat at the same time

When you do strength training with a ketogenic diet, the weight loss is due to body fat (adipose tissue), not muscle mass. Many people find it difficult to lose weight because they are losing muscle mass and body fat, which is not suitable for overall health. However, because this diet encourages protein consumption at every meal, as well as healthy fats, your amino acid intake will be sufficient to preserve your muscles without inhibiting your weight loss.

Foods Allowed

Here is the list of foods you can eat during the ketogenic diet:

1. Meat, poultry, fish, shellfish, and eggs from pasture-fed animals (animals are fed a grass-fed diet)
2. Fish and seafood caught in the wild
3. Eggs from pastured hens
4. Vegetables, including root vegetables such as beets and carrots and leafy greens such as spinach and kale.

5. Healthy fats such as coconut oil or olive oil that can be used in place of butter or other oils (11 grams per day maximum)

6. Nuts and seeds such as macadamia nuts, walnuts, and pumpkin seeds

7. Low to moderate amounts of dairy products such as yogurt and cheese

8. Non-starchy vegetables such as broccoli, cauliflower, and other cruciferous vegetables

9. Fruits

Foods That Are Not Allowed

Foods that are not allowed

When following the keto diet, you will want to avoid eating the following foods:

1. Grains including wheat, oats, rice, and corn

2. Sugar, including honey, maple syrup, and sugar in all its forms

3. Vegetable oils such as canola, sunflower, and soybean oil

4. Trans fats such as margarine and vegetable shortening

5. Juices and sugary drinks such as soda, fruit juices with added sugar or artificial sweeteners, or milk alternatives made with grains such as almond milk

6. Grain-based dairy products such as butter and yogurt

7. Legumes such as beans, soybeans, and peanuts

8. Starchy vegetables such as potatoes, peas, and corn

9. Processed foods of any kind, including sauces and any food that contains a high percentage of preservatives

10. Beer (pure alcohol)

11. Low-fat or nonfat dairy products such as yogurt and cheese (dairy products that are low in fat but have carbohydrates)

12. Fruit juices with added sugars or artificial sweeteners

Volume (liquid)

US Customary	Metric
1/8 teaspoon	.6 ml
1/4 teaspoon	1.2 ml
1/2 teaspoon	2.5 ml
3/4 teaspoon	3.7 ml
1 teaspoon	5 ml
1 tablespoon	15 ml
2 tablespoon or 1 fluid ounce	30 ml
1/4 cup or 2 fluid ounces	59 ml
1/3 cup	79 ml
1/2 cup	118 ml
2/3 cup	158 ml
3/4 cup	177 ml
1 cup or 8 fluid ounces	237 ml
2 cups or 1 pint	473 ml
4 cups or 1 quart	946 ml
8 cups or 1/2 gallon	1.9 liters
1 gallon	3.8 liters

Weight (mass)

US contemporary (ounces)	Metric (grams)
1/2 ounce	14 grams
1 ounce	28 grams
3 ounces	85 grams
3.53 ounces	100 grams
4 ounces	113 grams
8 ounces	227 grams
12 ounces	340 grams
16 ounces or 1 pound	454 grams

Volume Equivalents (liquid)*

3 teaspoons	1 tablespoon	0.5 fluid ounce
2 tablespoons	1/8 cup	1 fluid ounce
4 tablespoons	1/4 cup	2 fluid ounces
5 1/3 tablespoons	1/3 cup	2.7 fluid ounces
8 tablespoons	1/2 cup	4 fluid ounces
12 tablespoons	3/4 cup	6 fluid ounces
16 tablespoons	1 cup	8 fluid ounces
2 cups	1 pint	16 fluid ounces

BREAKFAST RECIPES

1. Sausage Biscuits and Gravy Breakfast Chaffle

Preparation Time: 10 minutes

Cooking Time: 20 minutes

Servings: 4

Ingredients

- Egg: 2
- Mozzarella cheese: 1 cup
- Onion: ¼ tbsp (granulated)
- Garlic: ¼ tbsp (granulated)
- Butter: 2 tbsp
- Garlic: 1 tbsp (finely minced)
- Almond flour: 1 tbsp
- Cornbread starch: 10 drops
- Baking powder: 1 tsp
- Dried parsley: 1 tsp
- Keto sausage biscuit and gravy: 1 batch

Directions

1. Preheat a mini waffle maker if needed and grease it
2. In a mixing bowl, beat eggs and add all the chaffle ingredients except the last one and mix well

3. Pour the mixture to the lower plate of the waffle maker and spread it evenly to cover the plate properly
4. Cook for at least 4 minutes to get the desired crunch
5. Remove the chaffle from the heat and keep aside
6. Make as many chaffles as your mixture and waffle maker allow
7. Prepare Sausage Gravy recipe and serve with yummy chaffles

Nutrition:

- calories 523 kcal
- fat 18 g
- carbs 7 g
- protein 3 g

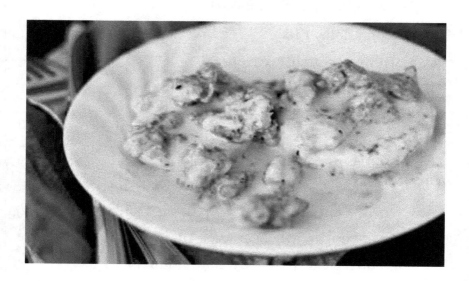

2. Bagel Chaffles With Peanut Butter

Preparation Time: 5 minutes

Cooking Time: 10 minutes

Servings: 2

Ingredients

- Eggs: 1
- Mozzarella cheese: ½ cup shredded
- Coconut flour: 1 tsp
- Everything Bagel seasoning: 1 tsp
- For the filling:
- Peanut butter: 3 tbsp
- Butter: 1 tbsp
- Powdered sweetener: 2 tbsp

Directions

1. Add all the chaffle ingredients in a bowl and whisk
2. Preheat your mini waffle iron if needed and grease it
3. Cook your mixture in the mini waffle iron for at least 4 minutes
4. Make as many chaffles as you can
5. Mix the filling ingredients together
6. When chaffles cool down, spread peanut butter

Nutrition:

- calories 523 kcal
- fat 18 g
- carbs 7 g
- protein 3 g

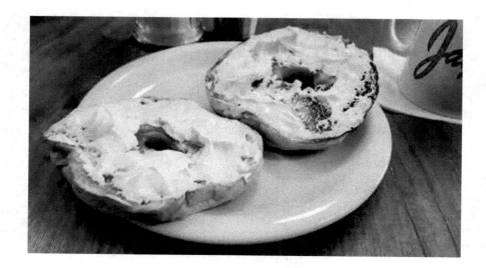

3. Gingerbread Chaffle

Preparation Time: 5 minutes

Cooking Time: 10 minutes

Servings: 2

Ingredients

- Egg: 1
- Mozzarella Cheese: ½ cup (shredded)
- Ginger: ½ tsp ground
- Erythritol: 1 tsp powdered
- Ground cinnamon: ½ tsp
- Ground nutmeg: ¼ tsp
- Ground cloves: 1/8 tsp
- Almond flour: 2 tbsp
- Baking powder: ½ tsp

Directions

1. Mix all the ingredients well together
2. Pour a layer on a preheated waffle iron
3. Cook the chaffle for around 5 minutes
4. Make as many chaffles as your mixture and waffle maker allow
5. Serve with your favorite topping

Nutrition:

- calories 523 kcal
- fat 18 g
- carbs 7 g
- protein 3 g

4. Lemon Almonds Chaffle

Preparation Time: 15 minutes

Cooking Time: 20 minutes

Servings: 4

Ingredients

- Cheddar cheese: 1/3 cup
- Egg: 1
- Lemon juice: 2 tbsp
- Almond flour: 2 tbsp
- Baking powder: 1/4 teaspoon
- Ground almonds: 2 tbsp
- Mozzarella cheese: 1/3 cup

Directions

1. Mix cheddar cheese, egg, lemon juice, almond flour, almond ground, and baking powder together in a bowl
2. Preheat your waffle iron and grease it
3. In your mini waffle iron, shred half of the mozzarella cheese
4. Add the mixture to your mini waffle iron
5. Again, shred the remaining mozzarella cheese on the mixture
6. Cook till the desired crisp is achieved

7. Make as many chaffles as your mixture and waffle maker allow

Nutrition:

- calories 523 kcal
- fat 18 g
- carbs 7 g
- protein 3 g

5. Mushroom Stuffed Chaffles

Preparation Time: 15 minutes

Cooking Time: 40 minutes

Servings: 2

Ingredients

- For Chaffle:
- Egg: 2
- Mozzarella Cheese: ½ cup (shredded)
- Onion powder: ½ tsp
- Garlic powder: ¼ tsp
- Salt: ¼ tsp or as per your taste
- Black pepper: ¼ tsp or as per your taste
- Dried poultry seasoning: ½ tsp
- For Stuffing:
- Onion: 1 small diced
- Mushrooms: 4 oz.
- Celery stalks: 3
- Butter: 4 tbsp
- Eggs: 3

Directions

1. Preheat a mini waffle maker if needed and grease it
2. In a mixing bowl, add all the chaffle ingredients and mix them well

3. Pour the mixture to the lower plate of the waffle maker and spread it evenly to cover the plate properly and close the lid
4. Cook for at least 4 minutes to get the desired crunch
5. Remove the chaffle from the heat and keep aside
6. Make as many chaffles as your mixture and waffle maker allow
7. Take a small frying pan and melt butter in it on medium-low heat
8. Sauté celery, onion, and mushrooms to make them soft
9. Take another bowl and tear chaffles down into minute pieces
10. Add the eggs and the veggies to it
11. Take a casserole dish, and add this new stuffing mixture to it
12. Bake it at 350 degrees for around 30 minutes and serve hot

Nutrition:

- calories 523
- fat 18 g
- carbs 7 g
- protein 3 g

6. Minty Mini Chaffles

Preparation Time: 5 minutes

Cooking Time: 10 minutes

Servings: 2

Ingredients

- Eggs: 2
- Mozzarella: 1 cup shredded
- Cream cheese: 2 tbsp
- Mint: ¼ cup chopped
- Almond flour: 2 tbsp
- Baking powder: ¾ tbsp
- Water: 2 tbsp (optional)

Directions

1. Preheat your mini waffle iron if needed
2. Mix all the above-mentioned ingredients in a bowl
3. Grease your waffle iron lightly
4. Cook your mixture in the mini waffle iron for at least 4 minutes or till the desired crisp is achieved and serve hot
5. Make as many chaffles as your mixture and waffle maker allow

Nutrition:

- calories 523 kcal
- fat 18 g
- carbs 7 g
- protein 3 g

7. Creamy Cinnamon Chaffles

Preparation Time: 5 minutes

Cooking Time: 10 minutes

Servings: 2

Ingredients

- Eggs: 2
- Shredded mozzarella: 1 cup
- Cream cheese: 2 tbsp
- Cinnamon powder: 1 tbsp
- Almond flour: 2 tbsp
- Baking powder: ¾ tbsp
- Water: 2 tbsp (optional)

Directions

1. Preheat your mini waffle iron if needed
2. Mix all the above-mentioned ingredients in a bowl
3. Grease your waffle iron lightly
4. Cook your mixture in the mini waffle iron for at least 4 minutes or till the desired crisp is achieved and serve hot
5. Make as many chaffles as your mixture and waffle maker allow

Nutrition:

- calories 523 kcal
- fat 18 g
- carbs 7 g
- protein 3 g

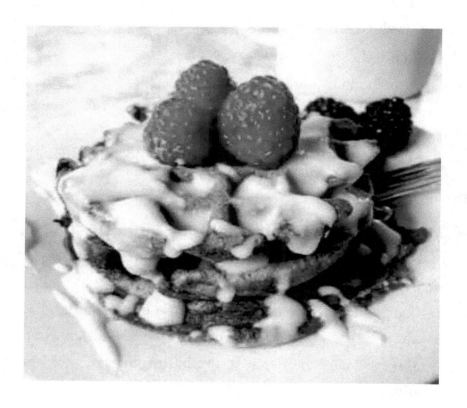

8. Hot Ham Chaffles

Preparation Time: 5 minutes

Cooking Time: 10 minutes

Servings: 2

Ingredients

- Eggs: 1
- Swiss cheese: 1 cup shredded
- Deli ham: ¼ cup chopped
- Mayonnaise: 1 tbsp
- Dijon mustard: 2 tsp
- Garlic salt: 1 tsp

Directions

1. Preheat your mini waffle iron if needed and grease it
2. Add egg, cheese, garlic salt, and ham a bowl and whisk
3. Cook your mixture in the mini waffle iron for at least 4 minutes
4. Make as many chaffles as your mixture and waffle maker allow
5. Combine together Dijon mustard and mayonnaise and serve with the dip

Nutrition:

- calories 523 kcal
- fat 18 g
- carbs 7 g
- protein 3 g

LUNCH RECIPES

9. Pumpkin Spice Chaffles

Preparation Time: 30 minutes

Cooking Time: 14 Minutes

Servings: 2

Ingredients:

- 1 egg, beaten
- ½ tsp. pumpkin pie spice
- ½ cup finely grated Mozzarella cheese
- 1 tbsp. sugar-free pumpkin puree

Directions:

1. Preheat the waffle iron.
2. In a medium bowl, mix all the ingredients.
3. Open the iron, pour in half of the batter, close, and cooking until crispy, 6 to 7 minutes.
4. Remove the chaffle onto a plate and set aside.
5. Make another chaffle with the remaining batter.
6. Allow cooling and serve afterward.

Nutrition:

- Kcal 468
- Fat 38g
- Net Carbs 2g
- Protein 26g

10. Open-faced Ham & Green Bell Pepper Chaffle Sandwich

Preparation Time: 20 minutes

Cooking Time: 10 Minutes

Servings: 2

Ingredients:

- 2 slices ham
- Cooking spray
- 1 green bell pepper, sliced into strips
- 2 slices cheese
- 1 tablespoon black olives, pitted and sliced
- 2 basic chaffles

Directions:

1. Cooking the ham in a pan coated with oil over medium heat.
2. Next, cooking the bell pepper.
3. Assemble the open-faced sandwich by topping each chaffle with ham and cheese, bell pepper and olives.
4. Toast in the oven until the cheese has melted a little.

Nutrition:

- Kcal 340
- Fat 30.2g
- Net Carbs 3.1g
- Protein 15g

11.   Lt. Chaffle Sandwich

Preparation Time: 20 minutes

Cooking Time: 15 Minutes

Servings: 2

Ingredients:

- Cooking spray
- 4 slices bacon
- 1 tablespoon mayonnaise
- 4 basic chaffles
- 2 lettuce leaves
- 2 tomato slices

Directions:

1. Coat your pan with foil and place it over medium heat.
2. Cooking the bacon until golden and crispy.
3. Spread mayo on top of the chaffle.
4. Top with the lettuce, bacon and tomato.
5. Top with another chaffle.

Nutrition:

- Kcal 398
- Fat 32g
- Net Carbs 4g
- Protein 24g

12. Mozzarella Peanut Chaffle

Preparation Time: 20 minutes

Cooking Time: 15 Minutes

Servings: 2

Ingredients:

- 1 egg, lightly beaten
- 2 tbsp. peanut butter
- 2 tbsp. Swerve
- 1/2 cup Mozzarella cheese, shredded

Directions:

1. Preheat your waffle maker.
2. In a bowl, mix egg, cheese, Swerve, and peanut butter until well combined.
3. Spray waffle maker with cooking spray.
4. Pour half batter in the hot waffle maker and cooking for minutes or until golden brown. Repeat with the remaining batter.
5. Serve and enjoy.

Nutrition:

- Calories: 515 kcal
- Fat 34.2g
- Net Carbs 7.3g
- Protein 50.8g

13. Cinnamon and Vanilla Chaffle

Preparation Time: 10 minutes

Cooking Time: 7–9 Minutes

Servings: 4

Ingredients:

- Batter
- 4 eggs
- 4 ounces sour cream
- 1 teaspoon vanilla extract
- 1 teaspoon cinnamon
- ¼ cup stevia
- 5 tablespoons coconut flour
- Other
- 2 tablespoons coconut oil to brush the waffle maker
- ½ teaspoon cinnamon for garnishing the chaffles

Directions:

1. Preheat the waffle maker.
2. Add the eggs and sour cream to a bowl and stir with a wire whisk until just combined.
3. Add the vanilla extract, cinnamon, and stevia and mix until combined.
4. Stir in the coconut flour and stir until combined.
5. Brush the heated waffle maker with coconut oil and add a few tablespoons of the batter.

6. Close the lid and cooking for about 7–8 minutes depending on your waffle maker.
7. Serve and enjoy.

Nutrition:

- Calories: 430 kcal
- Fat 23g
- Net Carbs 3g
- Protein 33g

14. Choco Chip Pumpkin Chaffle

Preparation Time: 20 minutes

Cooking Time: 15 Minutes

Servings: 2

Ingredients:

- 1 egg, lightly beaten
- 1 tbsp. almond flour
- 1 tbsp. unsweetened chocolate chips
- 1/4 tsp. pumpkin pie spice
- 2 tbsp. Swerve
- 1 tbsp. pumpkin puree
- 1/2 cup Mozzarella cheese, shredded

Directions:

1. Preheat your waffle maker.
2. In a small bowl, mix egg and pumpkin puree.
3. Add pumpkin pie spice, Swerve, almond flour, and cheese and mix well.
4. Stir in chocolate chips.
5. Spray waffle maker with cooking spray.
6. Pour half batter in the hot waffle maker and cooking for 4 minutes. Repeat with the remaining batter.
7. Serve and enjoy.

Nutrition:

- Calories: 453 kcal
- Fat: 31g
- Net Carbs: 6g
- Protein: 43g

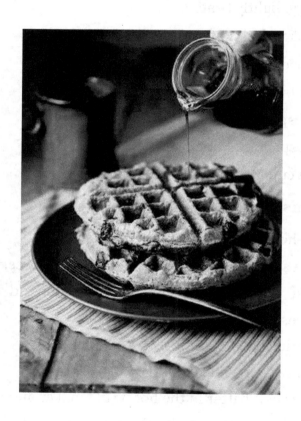

15. Sausage & Pepperoni Chaffle Sandwich

Preparation Time: 15 minutes

Cooking Time: 10 Minutes

Servings: 4

Ingredients:

- Cooking spray
- 2 cervelat sausage, sliced into rounds
- 12 pieces pepperoni
- 6 mushroom slices
- 4 teaspoons mayonnaise
- 4 big white onion rings
- 4 basic chaffles

Directions:

1. Spray your skillet with oil.
2. Place over medium heat.
3. Cooking the sausage until brown on both sides.
4. Transfer on a plate.
5. Cooking the pepperoni and mushrooms for 2 minutes.
6. Spread mayo on top of the chaffle.
7. Top with the sausage, pepperoni, mushrooms and onion rings.
8. Top with another chaffle.

Nutrition:

- Calories: 452 kcal
- Fat 36.4g
- Net Carbs 4g
- Protein 24g

16. Pizza Flavored Chaffle

Preparation Time: 15 minutes

Cooking Time: 12 Minutes

Servings: 3

Ingredients:

- 1 egg, beaten
- ½ cup cheddar cheese, shredded
- 2 tablespoons pepperoni, chopped
- 1 tablespoon keto marinara sauce
- 4 tablespoons almond flour
- 1 teaspoon baking powder
- ½ teaspoon dried Italian seasoning
- Parmesan cheese, grated

Directions:

1. Preheat your waffle maker.
2. In a bowl, mix the egg, cheddar cheese, pepperoni, marinara sauce, almond flour, baking powder and Italian seasoning.
3. Add the mixture to the waffle maker.
4. Close the device and cooking for minutes.
5. Open it and transfer chaffle to a plate.
6. Let cool for 2 minutes.
7. Repeat the steps with the remaining batter.
8. Top with the grated Parmesan and serve.

Nutrition:

- Calories: 485 kcal
- Fat 35g
- Net Carbs 2g
- Protein 26g

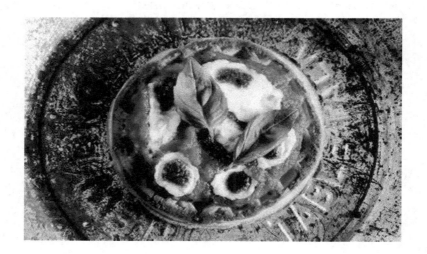

DINNER RECIPES

17. Chicken Green Butter Chaffles

Preparation Time: 10 minutes

Cooking Time: 25 minutes

Servings: 4

Ingredients:

- Chicken: 1/3 cup boiled and shredded
- Cabbage: 1/3 cup
- Broccoli: 1/3 cup
- Zucchini: 1/3 cup
- Egg: 2
- Mozzarella Cheese: 1 cup (shredded)
- Butter: 1 tbsp.
- Almond flour: 2 tbsp.
- Baking powder: ¼ tsp.
- Onion powder: a pinch
- Garlic powder: a pinch
- Salt: a pinch

Directions:

1. In a deep saucepan, boil cabbage, broccoli, and zucchini for five minutes or till they tender, then strain, and blend
2. Mix all the remaining ingredients well together

3. Pour a thin layer of the mixture on a preheated waffle iron
4. Add a layer of the blended vegetables on the mixture
5. Again, add more mixture over the top
6. Cooking the chaffle for around 5 minutes
7. Serve with your favorite sauce

Nutrition:

- Calories: 319 kcal
- Fat: 24 g
- Net Carbohydrates: 1 g
- Protein: 25 g

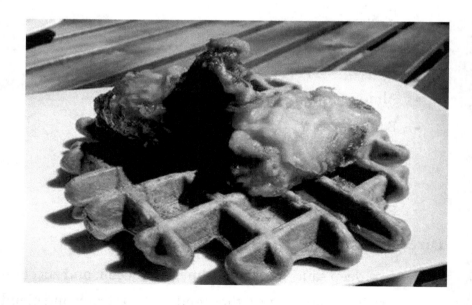

18.   Artichoke and Spinach Chicken Chaffle

Preparation Time: 10 minutes

Cooking Time: 25 minutes

Servings: 2

Ingredients:

- Chicken: 1/3 cup cooked and diced
- Spinach: 1/2 cup cooked and chopped
- Artichokes: 1/3 cup chopped
- Egg: 1
- Mozzarella Cheese: 1/3 cup (shredded)
- Cream cheese: 1 ounce
- Garlic powder: ¼ tsp.

Directions:

1. Preheat a mini waffle maker if needed and grease it
2. In a mixing bowl, add all the ingredients
3. Mix them all well
4. Pour the mixture to the lower plate of the waffle maker and spread it evenly to cover the plate properly
5. Close the lid
6. Cooking for at least 4 minutes to get the desired crunch
7. Remove the chaffle from the heat and keep aside for around one minute
8. Make as many chaffles as your mixture and waffle maker allow

9. Serve hot and enjoy!

Nutrition:

- Calories: 320 kcal
- Fat: 24 g
- Net Carbohydrates: 2 g
- Protein: 24 g

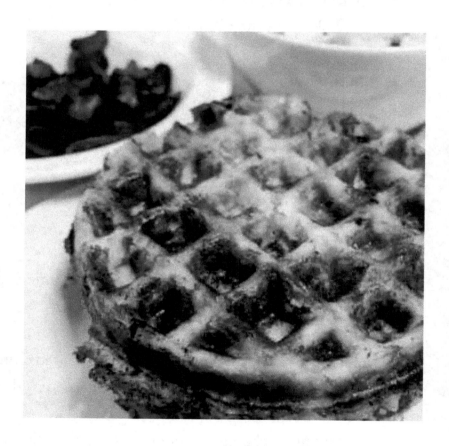

19. Boiled Chicken Halloumi Chaffle

Preparation Time: 15 minutes

Cooking Time: 20 minutes

Servings: 2

Ingredients:

- Boiled chicken: 1 cup shredded
- Pepper: ½ tsp.
- Salt: a pinch
- Halloumi cheese: 3 oz.
- Oregano: 1 tbsp.

Directions:

1. Take a bowl and add chicken, pepper, and salt
2. Make ½ inch thick slices of Halloumi cheese and divide each further into two
3. Put one slice of cheese in the unheated waffle maker and spread chicken on it
4. Top with another cheese slice and sprinkle oregano
5. Cooking the cheese for over 4-6 minutes till it turns golden brown
6. Remove from heat when a bit cool and serve with your favorite sauce

Nutrition:

- Calories: 843 kcal
- Total Fat: 65g
- Saturated Fat: 14g
- Protein: 59g
- Cholesterol: 156mg
- Carbohydrates: 6g
- Fiber: 1g
- Net Carbs: 5g

20. Aromatic Chicken Chaffles

Preparation Time: 10 minutes

Cooking Time: 40 minutes

Servings: 4

Ingredients:

- Chicken: 2 leg pieces
- Dried bay leaves: 1
- Cardamom: 1
- Whole black pepper: 4
- Clove: 4
- Water: 2 cups
- Eggs: 2
- Salt: ¼ tsp.
- Shredded mozzarella: 1 cup
- Baking powder: ¾ tbsp.

Directions:

1. Take a large pan and boil water in it
2. Add in chicken, bay leaves, black pepper, cloves, and cardamom and cover and boil for 20 minutes at least
3. Remove the chicken and shred finely and discard the bones
4. Preheat your mini waffle iron if needed
5. Mix all the remaining above-mentioned ingredients in a bowl and add in chicken

6. Grease your waffle iron lightly

7. Cooking your mixture in the mini waffle iron for at least 4 minutes or till the desired crisp is achieved and serve hot

8. Make as many chaffles as your mixture and waffle maker allows.

Nutrition:

- Calories: 1396 kcal
- Protein: 114.74 g
- Fat: 99.7 g
- Carbohydrates: 4.23 g

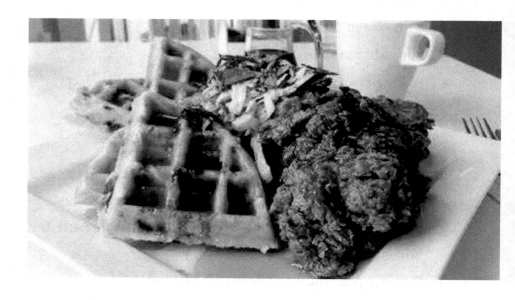

21. Pumpkin Chicken Chaffles

Preparation Time: 10 minutes

Cooking Time: 20 minutes

Servings: 2

Ingredients:

- Boiled chicken: ½ cup
- Pumpkin puree: ½ cup
- Pepper: ¼ tsp.
- Egg: 1
- Mozzarella Cheese: ½ cup (shredded)
- Almond flour: 2 tbsp.
- Onion powder: a pinch
- Garlic powder: a pinch
- Salt: as per your taste

Directions:

1. Mix all the ingredients well together in a bowl
2. Pour a layer of the mixture on a preheated waffle iron
3. Close the lid and cooking for 5 minutes
4. Serve with your favorite sauce

Nutrition:

- Calories: 865 kcal
- Protein: 60.23 g
- Fat: 64.07 g
- Carbohydrates: 9.88 g

22. Garlicky Chicken Pepper Chaffles

Preparation Time: 5 minutes

Cooking Time: 10 minutes

Servings: 2

Ingredients:

- Egg: 1
- Mozzarella cheese: ½ cup (shredded)
- Garlic cloves: 2 chopped
- Pepper: ½ cup finely chopped
- Chicken: ½ cup boiled and shredded
- Onion powder: 1 tsp.
- Salt and pepper: as per your taste

Directions:

1. Mix all the ingredients well together
2. Pour a layer on a preheated waffle iron
3. Cooking the chaffle for around 5 minutes
4. Make as many chaffles as your mixture and waffle maker allow

Nutrition:

- Calories: 210 kcal
- Fat: 9.3g
- Net Carbs: 1.3g
- Protein: 28.9g

23. Sliced Chicken Chaffles

Preparation Time: 15 minutes

Cooking Time: 25 minutes

Servings: 2

Ingredients:

- Egg: 2
- Mozzarella Cheese: 1½ cup (shredded)
- American cheese: 2 slices
- Chicken: 2 boneless slices
- Salt: ¼ tsp.
- Black pepper: ¼ tsp.
- Butter: 2 tbsp.

Directions:

1. Preheat a mini waffle maker if needed and grease it
2. In a mixing bowl, beat eggs and add shredded Mozzarella cheese and mix
3. Pour the mixture to the lower plate of the waffle maker and close the lid
4. Cooking for at least 4 minutes to get the desired crunch
5. Remove the chaffle from the heat
6. Add chicken, salt, and pepper together and mix
7. Fry the chicken in the butter from both sides till they turn golden

8. Place a cheese slice on the chicken immediately when removing from heat
9. Take two chaffles and put chicken and cheese in between
10. Make as many chaffles as your mixture and waffle maker allow
11. Serve hot and enjoy!

Nutrition:

- Calories: 268 kcal
- Fat: 20g
- Net Carbs: 3.5g
- Protein: 13.8g

24.   Ginger Chicken Cucumber Chaffle Roll

Preparation Time: 20 minutes

Cooking Time: 30 minutes

Servings: 2

Ingredients:

- For Garlic Chicken:
- Chicken mince: 1 cup
- Salt: ¼ tsp. or as per your taste
- Black pepper: ¼ tsp. or as per your taste
- Lemon juice: 1 tbsp.
- Butter: 2 tbsp.
- Garlic juvenile: 2 tbsp.
- Garlic powder: 1 tsp.
- Soy sauce: 1 tbsp.
- For Chaffle:
- Egg: 2
- Mozzarella cheese: 1 cup (shredded)
- Garlic powder: 1 tsp.
- For Serving:
- Cucumber: ½ cup (diced)
- Parsley: 1 tbsp.

Directions:

1. In a frying pan, melt butter and add juvenile garlic and sauté for 1 minute

2. Now add chicken mince and cooking till it tenders
3. When done, add rest of the ingredients and set aside
4. In a mixing bowl, beat eggs and add Mozzarella cheese to them with garlic powder
5. Mix them all well and pour to the greasy mini waffle maker
6. Cooking for at least 4 minutes to get the desired crunch
7. Remove the chaffle from the heat, add the chicken mixture in between with cucumber and fold
8. Make as many chaffles as your mixture and waffle maker allow
9. Serve hot and top with parsley

Nutrition:

- Calories: 156 kcal
- Fat: 6g
- Net Carbs: 5g
- Protein: 8g

APPETIZER RECIPES

25. Savory Cheddar Chaffles

Preparation Time: 5 minutes

Cooking Time: 8 minutes

Servings: 2

Ingredients:

- 1 large organic egg, beaten
- ½ cup Cheddar cheese, shredded
- Pinch of salt and freshly ground black pepper

Directions:

1. Preheat a mini waffle iron and then grease it.
2. In a bowl, place all the ingredients and beat until well combined.
3. Place half of the mixture into preheated waffle iron and cook for about 3-4 minutes or until golden brown.
4. Repeat with the remaining mixture.
5. Serve warm.

Nutrition:

- Calories: 150 kcal
- Net Carb: 0.6g
- Fat: 11.9g

- Carbohydrates: 0.6g
- Dietary Fiber: 0g
- Sugar: 0.3g
- Protein: 10.2g

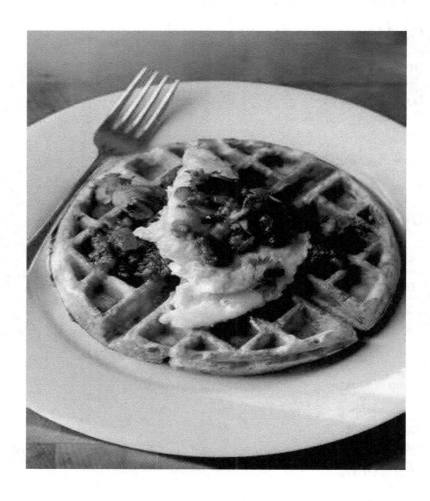

26. 2-Cheese Chaffles

Preparation Time: 10 minutes

Cooking Time: 8 minutes

Servings: 2

Ingredients:

- 1 organic egg white
- ¼ cup sharp cheddar cheese, shredded
- ¼ cup Monterey jack cheese, shredded
- ¾ teaspoon water
- 1 teaspoon coconut flour
- ¼ teaspoon organic baking powder
- 1/8 teaspoon red chili powder
- Pinch of salt

Directions:

1. Preheat a mini waffle iron and then grease it.
2. In a bowl, place all the ingredients and beat until well combined.
3. Place half of the mixture into preheated waffle iron and cook for about 4 minutes or until golden brown.
4. Repeat with the remaining mixture.
5. Serve warm.

Nutrition:

- Calories: 124 kcal
- Net Carb: 1g
- Fat: 9.2g
- Carbohydrates: 1.6g
- Dietary Fiber: 0.6g
- Sugar: 0.3g
- Protein: 9g

27.   Cheddar & Sour Cream Chaffles

Preparation Time: 10 minutes

Cooking Time: 32 minutes

Servings: 8

Ingredients:

- 3 organic eggs
- 1 cup cheddar cheese, shredded
- ¼ cup sour cream
- ¼ cup unflavored whey protein powder
- ½ teaspoon organic baking powder
- Pinch of salt

Directions:

1. Preheat a mini waffle iron and then grease it.
2. In a bowl, place all the ingredients and beat until well combined.
3. Divide the mixture into 8 portions.
4. Place 1 portion of the mixture into preheated waffle iron and cook for about 4 minutes or until golden brown.
5. Repeat with the remaining mixture.
6. Serve warm.

Nutrition:

- Calories: 110 kcal
- Net Carb: 1g
- Fat: 8g
- Carbohydrates: 1g
- Dietary Fiber: 0g
- Sugar: 0.4g
- Protein: 8.6g

28. Savory Cheddar & Psyllium Husk Chaffles

Preparation Time: 10 minutes

Cooking Time: 8 minutes

Servings: 2

Ingredients:

- 1 medium organic egg
- ¾ cup cheddar cheese, shredded
- 1 teaspoon psyllium husk
- Dash of hot sauce
- Pinch of salt and freshly ground black pepper

Directions:

1. Preheat a mini waffle iron and then grease it.
2. In a bowl, place all the ingredients and beat until well combined.
3. Place half of the mixture into preheated waffle iron and cook for about 4 minutes or until golden brown.
4. Repeat with the remaining mixture.
5. Serve warm.

Nutrition:

- Calories: 205 kcal
- Net Carb: 0.8g
- Fat: 16.2g
- Carbohydrates: 1.6g
- Dietary Fiber: 0.8g
- Sugar: 0.4g
- Protein: 13.3g

29. <u>Savory Heavy Cream Chaffles</u>

Preparation Time: 5 minutes

Cooking Time: 16 minutes

Servings: 4

Ingredients:

- 3 organic eggs
- 2 tablespoons heavy cream
- ¼ teaspoon organic baking powder
- 2 tablespoons coconut flour
- Pinch of salt and freshly ground black pepper

Directions:

1. Preheat a mini waffle iron and then grease it.
2. In a bowl, place all the ingredients and beat until well combined.
3. Place ¼ of the mixture into preheated waffle iron and cook for about 4 minutes or until golden brown.
4. Repeat with the remaining mixture.
5. Serve warm.

Nutrition:

- Calories: 88 kcal
- Net Carb: 1.6g
- Fat: 6.4g
- Carbohydrates: 3.1g
- Dietary Fiber: 1.5g
- Sugar: 0.3g
- Protein: 4.8g

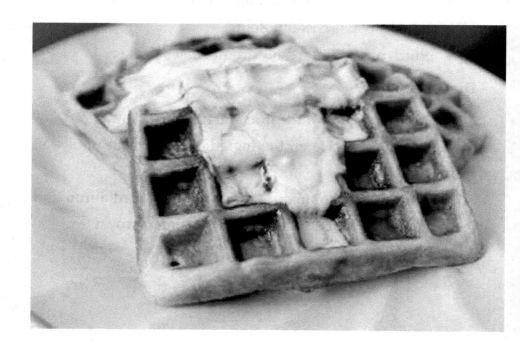

30. Garlic & Onion Powder Chaffles

Preparation Time: 5 minutes

Cooking Time: 5 minutes

Serving: 1

Ingredients:

- 1 organic egg, beaten
- ¼ cup Cheddar cheese, shredded
- 2 tablespoons almond flour
- ½ teaspoon organic baking powder
- ¼ teaspoon garlic powder
- ¼ teaspoon onion powder
- Pinch of salt

Directions:

1. Preheat a waffle iron and then grease it.
2. In a bowl, place all the ingredients and beat until well combined.
3. Place the mixture into preheated waffle iron and cook for about 3-5 minutes or until golden brown.
4. Serve warm.

Nutrition:

- Calories: 274 kcal
- Net Carb: 3.3g
- Fat: 21.3g
- Carbohydrates: 5g
- Dietary Fiber: 1.7g
- Sugar: 1.4g
- Protein: 12.8g

31. Garlic Powder & Oregano Chaffles

Preparation Time: 5 minutes

Cooking Time: 10 minutes

Servings: 2

Ingredients:

- ½ cup Mozzarella cheese, grated
- 1 medium organic egg, beaten
- 2 tablespoons almond flour
- ½ teaspoon dried oregano, crushed
- ½ teaspoon garlic powder
- Salt, to taste

Directions:

1. Preheat a mini waffle iron and then grease it.
2. In a medium bowl, place all ingredients and mix until well combined.
3. Place half of the mixture into preheated waffle iron and cook for about 4-5 minutes or until golden brown.
4. Repeat with the remaining mixture.
5. Serve warm.

Nutrition:

- Calories: 100 kcal
- Net Carb: 1.4g
- Fat: 7.2g
- Carbohydrates: 2.4g
- Dietary Fiber: 1g
- Sugar: 0.6g
- Protein: 4.9g

32. Garlic Powder & Italian Seasoning Chaffles

Preparation Time: 10 minutes

Cooking Time: 20 minutes

Servings: 4

Ingredients:

- 1 large organic egg, beaten
- ½ cup Mozzarella cheese, shredded
- ¼ cup Parmesan cheese, grated
- 1 teaspoon Italian seasoning
- ¼ teaspoon garlic powder

Directions:

1. Preheat a mini waffle iron and then grease it.
2. In a medium bowl, place all ingredients and mix until well combined.
3. Place ¼ of the mixture into preheated waffle iron and cook for about 3-5 minutes or until golden brown.
4. Repeat with the remaining mixture.
5. Serve warm.

Nutrition:

- Calories: 90 kcal
- Net Carb: 1.5g
- Fat: 6.1g
- Carbohydrates: 1.5g
- Dietary Fiber: 0g
- Sugar: 0.2g
- Protein: 8.4g

DESSERT RECIPES

33. Butter & Cream Cheese Chaffles

Preparation Time: 10 minutes

Cooking Time: 16 minutes

Servings: 4

Ingredients

- 2 tablespoons butter, melted and cooled
- 2 large organic eggs
- 2 ounces cream cheese, softened
- ¼ cup powdered erythritol
- 1½ teaspoons organic vanilla extract
- Pinch of salt
- ¼ cup almond flour
- 2 tablespoons coconut flour
- 1 teaspoon organic baking powder

Directions:

1. Preheat a mini waffle iron and then grease it.
2. In a bowl, add the butter and eggs and beat until creamy.
3. Add the cream cheese, erythritol, vanilla extract, and salt, and beat until well combined.
4. Add the flours and baking powder and beat until well combined.

5. Place ¼ of the mixture into preheated waffle iron and cook for about 4 minutes.
6. Repeat with the remaining mixture.
7. Serve warm.

Nutrition:

- Calories 217 kcal
- Net Carbs 3.3 g
- Total Fat 18 g
- Saturated Fat 8.8 g
- Cholesterol 124 mg
- Sodium 173 mg
- Total Carbs 6.6 g
- Fiber 3.3 g
- Sugar 1.2 g
- Protein 5.3 g

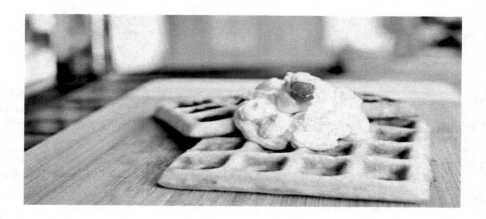

34. Cinnamon Chaffles

Preparation Time: 10 minutes

Cooking Time: 8 minutes

Servings: 2

Ingredients

- For Chaffles:
- 1 large organic egg, beaten
- ¾ cup mozzarella cheese, shredded
- ½ tablespoon unsalted butter, melted
- 2 tablespoons blanched almond flour
- 2 tablespoons erythritol
- ½ teaspoon ground cinnamon
- ½ teaspoon Psyllium husk powder
- ¼ teaspoon organic baking powder
- ½ teaspoon organic vanilla extract
- For Topping:
- 1 teaspoon powdered Erythritol
- ¾ teaspoon ground cinnamon

Directions:

1. Preheat a waffle iron and then grease it.
2. For chaffles: In a medium bowl, put all ingredients and with a fork, mix until well combined.
3. Place half of the mixture into preheated waffle iron and cook for about 3–5 minutes.

4. Repeat with the remaining mixture.
5. Meanwhile, for topping: in a small bowl, mix together the erythritol and cinnamon.
6. Place the chaffles onto serving plates and set aside to cool slightly.
7. Sprinkle with the cinnamon mixture and serve immediately.

Nutrition:

- Calories 142 kcal
- Net Carbs 2.1 g
- Total Fat 10.6 g
- Saturated Fat 4 g
- Cholesterol 106 mg
- Sodium 122 mg
- Total Carbs 4.1 g
- Fiber 2 g
- Sugar 0.3 g
- Protein 7.7 g

35. Layered Chaffles

Preparation Time: 5 minutes

Cooking Time: 10 minutes

Servings: 2

Ingredients

- 1 organic egg, beaten and divided
- ½ cup cheddar cheese, shredded and divided
- Pinch of salt

Directions:

1. Preheat a mini waffle iron and then grease it.
2. Place about 1/8 cup of cheese in the bottom of the waffle iron and top with half of the beaten egg.
3. Now, place 1/8 cup of cheese on top and cook for about 4–5 minutes.
4. Repeat with the remaining cheese and egg.
5. Serve warm.

Nutrition:

- Calories 145 kcal
- Net Carbs 0.5 g
- Total Fat 11.6 g
- Saturated Fat 6.6 g
- Cholesterol 112 mg
- Sodium 284 g
- Total Carbs 0.5 g
- Fiber 0 g
- Sugar 0.3 g
- Protein 9.8 g

36. Blueberry Cream Cheese Chaffles

Preparation Time: 10 minutes

Cooking Time: 8 minutes

Servings: 2

Ingredients

- 1 organic egg, beaten
- 1/3 cup mozzarella cheese, shredded
- 1 teaspoon cream cheese, softened
- 1 teaspoon coconut flour
- ¼ teaspoon organic baking powder
- ¾ teaspoon powdered erythritol
- ¼ teaspoon ground cinnamon
- ¼ teaspoon organic vanilla extract
- Pinch of salt
- 1 tablespoon fresh blueberries

Directions:

1. Preheat a mini waffle iron and then grease it.
2. In a bowl, place all ingredients except for blueberries and beat until well combined.
3. Fold in the blueberries.
4. Place half of the mixture into preheated waffle iron and cook for about 4 minutes.
5. Repeat with the remaining mixture.
6. Serve warm.

Nutrition:

- Calories 90 kcal
- Net Carbs 2.9 g
- Total Fat 5 g
- Saturated Fat 2.7 g
- Cholesterol 97 mg
- Sodium 161 mg
- Total Carbs 5.7 g
- Fiber 2.8 g
- Sugar 1.2 g
- Protein 5.7 g

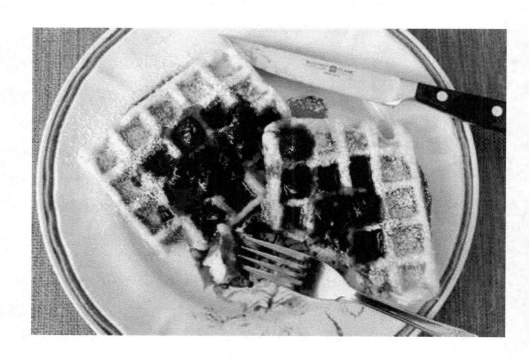

37. Raspberry Chaffles

Preparation Time: 10 minutes

Cooking Time: 8 minutes

Servings: 2

Ingredients

- 1 organic egg, beaten
- 1 tablespoon cream cheese, softened
- ½ cup mozzarella cheese, shredded
- 1 tablespoon powdered erythritol
- ¼ teaspoon organic raspberry extract
- ¼ teaspoon organic vanilla extract

Directions:

1. Preheat a mini waffle iron and then grease it.
2. In a medium bowl, put all ingredients and with a fork, mix until well combined.
3. Place half of the mixture into preheated waffle iron and cook for about 4 minutes.
4. Repeat with the remaining mixture.
5. Serve warm.

Nutrition:

- Calories 69 kcal
- Net Carbs 0.6 g
- Total Fat 5.2 g
- Saturated Fat 2.5 g
- Cholesterol 91 mg
- Sodium 88 mg
- Total Carbs 0.6 g
- Fiber 0 g
- Sugar 0.2 g
- Protein 5.2 g

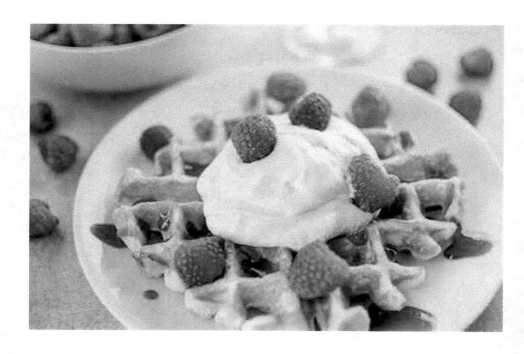

38. Red Velvet Chaffles

Preparation Time: 10 minutes

Cooking Time: 8 minutes

Servings: 2

Ingredients

- 2 tablespoons cacao powder
- 2 tablespoons erythritol
- 1 organic egg, beaten
- 2 drops super red food coloring
- ¼ teaspoon organic baking powder
- 1 tablespoon heavy whipping cream

Directions:

1. Preheat a mini waffle iron and then grease it.
2. In a medium bowl, put all ingredients and with a fork, mix until well combined.
3. Place half of the mixture into preheated waffle iron and cook for about 4 minutes.
4. Repeat with the remaining mixture.
5. Serve warm.

Nutrition:

- Calories 70 kcal
- Net Carbs 1.7 g
- Total Fat 6 g
- Saturated Fat 3 g
- Cholesterol 92 mg
- Sodium 34 mg
- Total Carbs 3.2 g
- Fiber 1.5 g
- Sugar 0.2 g
- Protein 3.9 g

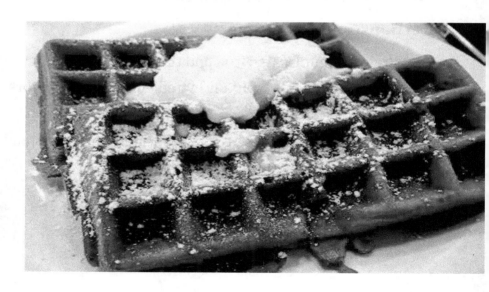

39. Walnut Pumpkin Chaffles

Preparation Time: 10 minutes

Cooking Time: 10 minutes

Servings: 2

Ingredients

- 1 organic egg, beaten
- ½ cup mozzarella cheese, shredded
- 2 tablespoons almond flour
- 1 tablespoon sugar-free pumpkin puree
- 1 teaspoon erythritol
- ¼ teaspoon ground cinnamon
- 2 tablespoons walnuts, toasted and chopped

Directions:

1. Preheat a mini waffle iron and then grease it.
2. In a bowl, add all ingredients except pecans and beat until well combined.
3. Fold in the walnuts.
4. Place half of the mixture into preheated waffle iron and cook for about 5 minutes.
5. Repeat with the remaining mixture.
6. Serve warm.

Nutrition:

- Calories 148 kcal
- Net Carbs 1.6 g
- Total Fat 11.8 g
- Saturated Fat 2 g
- Cholesterol 86 mg
- Sodium 74 mg
- Total Carbs 3.3 g
- Fiber 1.7 g
- Sugar 0.8 g
- Protein 6.7 g

40. Pumpkin Cream Cheese Chaffles

Preparation Time: 10 minutes

Cooking Time: 10 minutes

Servings: 2

Ingredients

- 1 organic egg, beaten
- ½ cup mozzarella cheese, shredded
- 1½ tablespoon sugar-free pumpkin puree
- 2 teaspoons heavy cream
- 1 teaspoon cream cheese, softened
- 1 tablespoon almond flour
- 1 tablespoon erythritol
- ½ teaspoon pumpkin pie spice
- ½ teaspoon organic baking powder
- 1 teaspoon organic vanilla extract

Directions:

1. Preheat a mini waffle iron and then grease it.
2. In a medium bowl, put all ingredients and with a fork, mix until well combined.
3. Place half of the mixture into preheated waffle iron and cook for about 3–5 minutes.
4. Repeat with the remaining mixture.
5. Serve warm.

Nutrition:

- Calories 110 kcal
- Net Carbs 2.5 g
- Total Fat 7.8 g
- Saturated Fat 3.1 g
- Cholesterol 94 mg
- Sodium 82 mg
- Total Carbs 3.3 g
- Fiber 0.8 g
- Sugar 1 g
- Protein 5.2 g

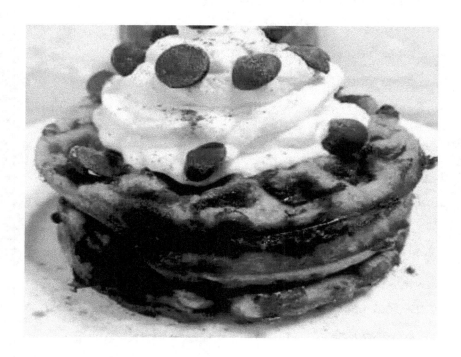

CONCLUSION

Chaffles is the amazing new invention you've been waiting for. It's a revolutionary, patent-pending, and 100% vegan protein bar with a thousand uses.

What are chaffles? Chaffles is a delicious new product that can be used to replace the high fat and high sugar snacks in your diet like cheese chips or chocolate bars. It's also gluten-free, vegan, non-GMO, low in sodium and preservative free! The best part is that chaffles taste just as good as candy! You'll never want anything else again after trying this life changing snack.

The combination of protein and savory chaffle taste will keep you wanting to eat more every time. Chaffles are also a great substitute for those times that you feel like having something sweet, but want something healthy with a lot of flavor.

Chaffles come in an assortment of flavors like Pecan Pie or Cherry Pie and can be served with a drizzle of your favorite nut butter or cinnamon sugar for an awesome snack. Or you can create your own combinations by mixing them up the way that makes your mouth water.

Chaffles are great for both kids and adults. They're the perfect snack to bring on a hike for an afternoon treat or to eat on a road trip or flights. Even better, they create a new way for parents to get their kids to eat protein without them even knowing what they're eating. Now if you want your children to enjoy healthy food without complaining, chaffles will be your best friend.

No matter what you eat chaffles with, it will never disappoint! Have it with chicken noodle soup or mashed potatoes for dinner or have it with salad at lunch.

Chaffle is a perfect combination for keto dieters. Besides, keto diet is always low in carbs and high in fat so chaffle is an amazing option for it.

Chaffles are very versatile and can be used as a spread for your favorite bagel or toast, or even on top of a pizza before baking it. You can also use chaffles as an ingredient for your own meals like pancakes, pies, donuts, breads and so much more!

Chaffle comes in two different flavors: savory and sweet. The savory flavor is more of a BBQ flavor while the sweet flavor is more cookie dough style. The savory chaffles are perfect for replacing things like bread and crackers, while sweet chaffles can be used as a dessert or drink! You can also add chaffle to your favorite dessert recipes for an amazing taste.

Chaffles are the most unique tasting protein bar around that is also good for you. You won't believe how good they taste until you try them for yourself. This incredible product is sure to revolutionize your snacking experience and change the way you think about eating healthy forever.

Always remember when making your own chaffle recipes, you can choose from almost any combination of things like fruits, cereals, nuts and seeds. You can even use different types of chocolate in some recipes. Anything goes with chaffle!

What's even more exciting is that chaffles come in many sizes to fit anyone's taste and diet.

It's time to ditch your unhealthy snacks for life changing chaffles!

CPSIA information can be obtained
at www.ICGtesting.com
Printed in the USA
LVHW022354270521
688666LV00034B/1185

9 781802 348699